What you really need to know about

CARING FOR SOMEONE AFTER A STROKE

Dr Robert Buckman

with Dr Jenny Sutcliffe

Introduced by John Cleese

MARSHALL PUBLISHING • LONDON

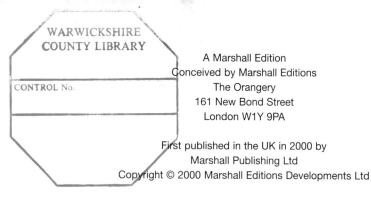

A Marshall Edition
Conceived by Marshall Editions
The Orangery
161 New Bond Street
London W1Y 9PA

First published in the UK in 2000 by
Marshall Publishing Ltd
Copyright © 2000 Marshall Editions Developments Ltd

ISBN: 1 84028 340 8

Originated in Italy by Articolor
Printed in and bound in Italy by Milanostampa

Project Editor Alison Murdoch
Additional Editing Jill Cropper
Indexer Stephen Fall
Designer Louise Morley
Illustrator Coral Mula
Picture Research Vickie Walters
Managing Editor Anne Yelland
Managing Art Editor Helen Spencer
Editorial Director Ellen Dupont
Art Director Dave Goodman
Editorial Coordinator Ros Highstead
Production Nikki Ingram, Anna Pauletti

Cover photography: front Denis Boissary/Telegraph Colour Library;
back Bluestone Productions/Telegraph Colour Library

The consultant for this book, Dr J. V. Bowler, is Consultant Neurologist
at London's Royal Free Hospital. He trained in stroke neurology at
Imperial College, London, and in the Department of Clinical Neurological Sciences,
University of Western Ontario, Canada.

Note: In this book we refer to the patient as 'he' or 'she' in alternate articles.
All the information is equally applicable to both men and women.

Contents

Foreword

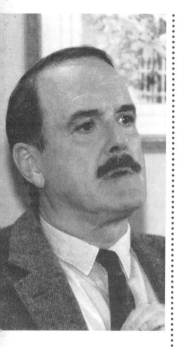

Most of you know me best as someone who makes people laugh.

But for 30 years I've also been involved with communicating information. And one particular area in which communication often breaks down is the doctor/patient relationship. We have all come across doctors who fail to communicate clearly, using complex medical terms when a simple explanation would do, and dismiss us with a "come back in a month if you still feel unwell". Fortunately I met Dr Robert Buckman.

Rob is one of North America's leading experts on cancer, but far more importantly he is a doctor who believes that hiding behind medical jargon is unhelpful and unprofessional. He wants his patients to understand what is wrong with them, and spends many hours with them—and their families and close friends—making sure they understand everything. Together we created a series of videos, with the jargon-free title Videos for Patients. Their success has prompted us to write books that explore medical conditions in the same clear, simple terms.

This book is one of a series that will tell you all you need to know, as a carer, about the causes, effects and treatment of stroke. It assumes nothing. If you have a helpful, honest, communicative doctor, you will find here the extra information that he or she simply may not have time to tell you. If you are less fortunate, this book will help to give you a much clearer picture of your situation.

More importantly—and this was a major factor in the success of the videos—you can access the information here again and again. Turn back, read over, until you really know what your doctor's diagnosis means. In addition, because in the middle of a consultation you may not think of everything you would like to ask your doctor, you can also use the book to help you formulate the questions you would like to discuss with him or her.

John Cleese

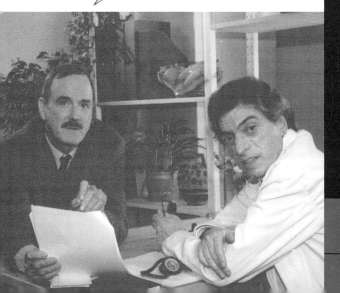

Introduction

Each year around 100,000 people in the UK have a stroke for the first time. The majority—more than 80 percent—survive, but many are left with varying degrees of physical or other incapacity. In fact, a stroke is the main cause of serious disability. But a stroke patient does not just have to contend with physical problems. There are often also problems with swallowing, speech and communication, while the shock of what has happened can cause anxiety and frustration. Later, this may turn to depression and anger. Nor is it only the stroke patient who suffers; his whole family—and his carer in particular—are affected by the change and turmoil that follow a stroke.

At first, the outlook can seem bleak. However, while pessimism may be understandable, it is not justified in the vast majority of cases. Though full recovery from a stroke is rare, most stroke patients regain a reasonable degree of independence. For example, two-thirds of those who cannot walk without help in the first days after a stroke do so within a year, and 90 percent of stroke patients regain the ability to feed themselves.

A positive approach

The extent to which a stroke patient recovers and regains independence, and how quickly, depends on a number of factors. Obviously, the severity of the stroke and the extent of the damage it causes play a part. But so too does the attitude and determination of both patient and carer. With a postive approach, based on an understanding of both the problems and possibilities, much can be achieved.

This book is designed to give carers—and patients—the knowledge not only to cope with the problems but to take advantage of the possibilities and promote recovery. It explains what a stroke is, what causes one and what the medical team does, both in the short term, in hospital, and in the longer term, in the patient's own home, as part of the rehabilitation programme. It shows carers how to help a stroke patient regain mobility, overcome communication problems, cope with emotional problems and regain independence.

Coping with caring

The road to recovery can be a long one for both carer and patient. Being a carer is demanding, both physically and emotionally, and some carers lose sight of their own needs. This helps neither the carer nor the patient. For this reason, the last section of this book addresses the needs of carers. It suggests practical ways to help carers cope and retain some control over their lives.

A considerable amount of support is available to carers, not just from family and friends, but from the social services and numerous voluntary organizations. This includes help with finances, social life and even respite care for holidays. This book tells you what support is available and how to obtain it.

FINDING OUT MORE

Caring for a stroke patient can be a demanding task, and a lack of information and help can make it even more difficult. Two specialist organizations can make an enormous difference to a carer's life—The Stroke Association and The Carers National Association. Details can be found on page 78.

Chapter

1

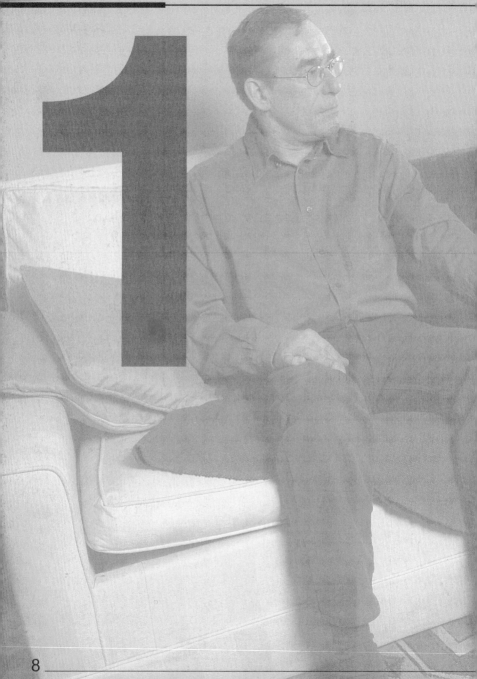

SYMPTOMS &
CAUSES

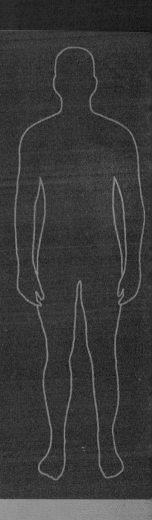

What is a stroke?

✓ 75 percent of strokes are caused by a blockage in an artery.

✓ Most others are caused by bleeding from a blood vessel into the surrounding tissues.

A stroke, also known as a cerebrovascular accident (CVA), happens when the blood supply to part of the brain is cut off. In about 75 percent of strokes, the cause is a blockage (clot) in one of the arteries that brings blood to the brain. The second main reason is a burst in the wall of a blood vessel, which allows blood to seep into the surrounding tissues (a haemorrhage). This increases the pressure on the brain, killing some of the cells, and stops tissues farther along the path of the burst vessel getting the blood they need to function healthily.

The blood supply to an area of the brain may also be disrupted for short periods of time, without causing a full-blown stroke. This can happen just once or repeatedly. If the symptoms last for less than 24 hours, it is known as

THE BRAIN'S BLOOD SUPPLY

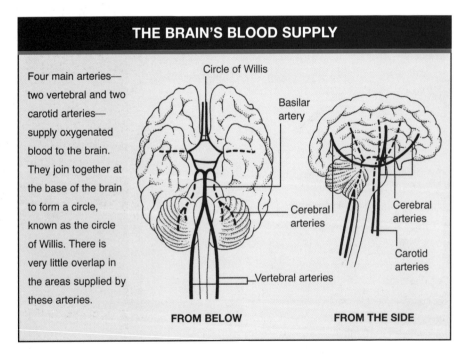

Four main arteries—two vertebral and two carotid arteries—supply oxygenated blood to the brain. They join together at the base of the brain to form a circle, known as the circle of Willis. There is very little overlap in the areas supplied by these arteries.

Circle of Willis

Basilar artery

Cerebral arteries

Vertebral arteries

Cerebral arteries

Carotid arteries

FROM BELOW

FROM THE SIDE

a transient ischaemic attack (TIA, see p. 14). However, doctors now know that any disruption of the blood supply that lasts for more than one hour can cause scarring of the brain and the definition of a TIA may change to reflect this.

The eyes receive their blood supply from the same vessels that supply the brain. TIAs can affect the blood supply to one eye, causing temporary loss of vision or blurring—called amaurosis fugax (AFx) or transient monocular blindness (TMB).

What damage does a stroke cause?

The effect a stroke has on the brain is much the same whatever its cause. When part of the brain is cut off from its blood supply, the cells are starved of oxygen and stop working. If the blood supply is not restored within about four minutes, the cells die (cerebral infarction). The physical and mental after-effects of a stroke depend on the part of the brain that is affected.

Separate parts of the brain work to control movement, speech and vision respectively. These control centres are made up of nerve cells (neurons), each of which has a specific function. For example, chains of interlinked neurons control every movement of the muscles.

Each neuron has three parts: dendrites, a cell body and an axon. The dendrites, which spread out like thin antlers, receive messages and pass them into the cell body. The cell body decides on what action to take and fires off orders through the axon to the next nerve cell. But if any part of this chain of command is interrupted, as can happen with a stroke when an area of cells dies, the whole neuron system fails, and the function it controls—such as speech or movement—is lost.

**YOU REALLY
NEED TO KNOW**

◆ Brain cells die if they are starved of oxygenated blood for longer than four minutes.

◆ In most cases of stroke, blood supply to the brain cells does not stop completely but continues at a reduced level. This makes treatment possible for up to several hours after the stroke.

◆ The effect of a stroke depends on the area of brain tissue damaged and its function before the stroke.

What is a stroke?

What causes a stroke?

The direct causes of a stroke are either a blocked artery or a haemorrhage, as a result of an artery wall bursting. Both have their own trigger factors, and these triggers are the indirect causes of a stroke.

What causes a blockage?

An artery can become completely or partially blocked by a thrombus (thrombosis) or an embolus (embolism). A thrombus is a clot of blood that usually forms in an artery already narrowed by a build-up of fatty matter (atherosclerosis), which has a reduced blood flow.

An embolus is an obstruction in the bloodstream— usually a small clot of blood that has broken away from a thrombus, but possibly a globule of fat or a bubble of air. Emboli usually form in the heart and in the arteries that take blood to the brain.

If the heart's muscular wall has already been damaged by a heart attack, blood clots may form inside and break off as emboli. If the heartbeat is irregular or weak, blood may flow so slowly in parts of the heart that it clots very easily, and this can cause emboli. There is about a 50 percent chance that an embolus that forms in the heart region will then be carried in the bloodstream to the brain.

Some emboli are too small to block an artery and so are carried deeper into the circulation of the brain until they block one of the smaller blood vessels that branch off the arteries (arterioles). When this happens, only a very small area of the brain may be affected and the damage may either not be noticed or be put down to ageing or the first signs of Alzheimer's disease. If an individual has atherosclerosis, more emboli are likely to develop, leading to a succession of very small strokes that cause gradual mental or physical deterioration.

What causes a haemorrhage?

In most cases of haemorrhage, the artery wall bursts when an individual's blood pressure suddenly rises in an area that has already been seriously weakened. For example, the wall may have been weakened by long-standing untreated high blood pressure.

Indirect causes

The major causes of both haemorrhage and blockage are general hardening of the arteries (arteriosclerosis) and atherosclerosis, making these the main indirect causes of strokes. Various factors make both these problems more likely to occur, including old age, an inherited predisposition, high blood pressure, diabetes, smoking and obesity.

WHO IS AT RISK?

Some people are more likely to have a stroke than others. Risk factors include:

◆ Age—incidence of arteriosclerosis increases with age
◆ Atherosclerosis
◆ Diabetes
◆ Heart disease
◆ High blood cholesterol
◆ High blood pressure
◆ High oestrogen levels—as in some contraceptive pills, hormone replacement therapy and prostate cancer drugs
◆ Gender—more men than women under 70 have strokes
◆ Transient ischaemic attacks—30 percent of those who suffer a TIA will have a stroke in the next three years

◆ A stroke caused by a haemorrhage occurs when a previously weakened arterial wall is subjected to a sudden rise in blood pressure.

◆ An artery may become blocked by a thrombus (a clot of blood) or an embolus, which is normally a small piece that has broken off a thrombus.

◆ The main causes of a blockage or a haemorrhage are arteriosclerosis and atherosclerosis.

What causes a stroke?

Types of stroke

✓ The carotid and cerebral arteries are the most commonly affected, followed by the basilar artery.

✓ Around 90 percent of strokes occur in the left or right cerebral hemispheres, which are responsible for thinking, movement and talking.

✓ Most of the remainder occur in the brain stem, which controls breathing and heartbeat. In a few cases, the cerebellum, which regulates balance and coordination, may be affected.

Doctors classify strokes in a variety of ways. The main categories used are:

◆ the cause of the stroke—haemorrhage, a thrombus or an embolus;

◆ the symptoms of the stroke—for example, language or swallowing difficulties or paralysis of one side of the body (hemiplegia);

◆ the area of the brain where the stroke has occurred;

◆ the artery or arterioles involved.

So, for example, a doctor might talk about a "left cerebral infarct", meaning a stroke in a branch of the left cerebral artery that has caused damage in the left cerebral hemisphere. This will, in fact, cause movement difficulties on the right side of the body. The effects of a stroke are always on the opposite side of the body to the damaged area of the brain because each side of the brain controls the opposite side of the body.

Transient ischaemic attacks

Strokes are also classified according to how long the symptoms last. When the symptoms persist for less than 24 hours, the stroke is called a transient ischaemic attack (TIA) or "mini-stroke".

TIAs, which can take the form of mild and temporary weakness, must always be taken seriously. They are warning signs that a stroke is possible—without treatment, around 30 percent of those who suffer a TIA are likely to have a major stroke within the next three years.

Multiple infarcts

In most strokes, a single event affects a nearby area of the brain. Multiple infarcts, although they are "true" strokes, are infrequent, irregular, small strokes that only affect tiny areas of the brain. Most of those who experience multiple infarcts are elderly people whose small blood vessels have become weakened by time. The symptoms of multiple infarcts—memory loss and confusion—are similar to those of senility or Alzheimer's disease until the deterioration gets more pronounced.

SUBARACHNOID HAEMORRHAGE

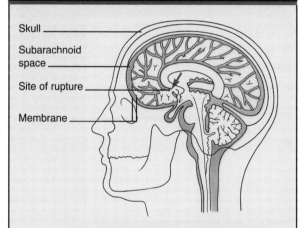

Skull
Subarachnoid space
Site of rupture
Membrane

When the wall of an artery bursts, the bleeding is not always into the brain tissue itself. In what is known as a subarachnoid haemorrhage, blood enters the space between two of the membranes lining the brain—the subarachnoid space. The usual cause is a burst aneurysm (a balloon-like swelling of the artery wall). This can result in damage to the brain and stroke-like symptoms. Emergency surgery may be needed to reduce the pressure on the brain, and tie off the burst blood vessel. Even with prompt treatment the outcome of a subarachnoid haemorrhage is often serious.

◆ Transient ischaemic attacks are important warnings that a more serious stroke may soon occur.

◆ Most of the risk of a stroke occurring after a TIA is within the first few weeks. The patient should be treated urgently.

◆ Strokes that begin with severe headache or loss of consciousness are more likely to be caused by a haemorrhage.

Types of stroke

Symptoms of a stroke

Stroke symptoms vary considerably, depending on which area of the brain is affected. In general terms, they can be divided into physical problems, mental problems and problems with language.

PHYSICAL AND MENTAL SYMPTOMS

PHYSICAL SYMPTOMS

◆ Loss of consciousness during the stroke—60 percent of strokes occur when the individual is awake. Loss of consciousness generally accompanies a stroke caused by a haemorrhage.

◆ Bowel and/or bladder incontinence—90 percent regain control after the first few weeks.

◆ Paralysis or weakness of the muscles—75 percent of people have an arm and leg affected on the same side of the body; smaller, more skilled movements, such as those required to write, are often experienced by those people who do not have full paralysis.

◆ Spasticity—tension in the muscles in the affected limbs— increases in the first few days or weeks after a stroke and the muscles may jerk involuntarily. This looks alarming at the time but improves the chance of eventual recovery.

◆ Involuntary jerking movements (reflex actions) of a paralyzed limb while using an unaffected limb.

◆ Loss of sensation in affected areas—around 30 percent experience mild loss of sensation and, rarely, there may be complete lack of feeling on one side of the body or a limb.

◆ Swallowing difficulties—swallowing involves a large number of nerves and muscles and about 30 percent find it difficult during the first few days.

It is rare for an individual to experience all the symptoms listed in the table below, and the severity of symptoms varies from mild and transient to severe and permanently disabling.

◆ Slurred speech (dysarthria)—resulting from weakness or paralysis of muscles.

◆ Sight problems—usually temporary; occasionally permanent.

◆ Loss of "righting reflexes", which maintain an individual's balance, and poor co-ordination both affect a person's posture and movement.

◆ General tiredness and lack of stamina.

MENTAL SYMPTOMS

◆ Confusion—this normally improves over the first few days.

◆ Loss of visual or verbal memory.

◆ Difficulties in learning and reasoning.

◆ Loss of concentration and organizing abilities.

◆ Psychological problems—initially anxiety and frustration, often followed by depression and anger.

LANGUAGE PROBLEMS

◆ There may be a number of different problems with language if the brain centre that controls language is affected by a stroke—in most people, this centre is in the left cerebral hemisphere.

◆ Motor dysphasia—patients understand language perfectly but cannot express themselves through speech or writing.

◆ Receptive dysphasia—patients can speak and write but find it difficult to understand what is said or written.

YOU REALLY NEED TO KNOW

◆ As well as causing physical and mental problems, a stroke may result in difficulties with language.

◆ The degree and type of symptoms depend on which part of the brain is affected and how much of it has been damaged.

◆ Very few people will suffer all the symptoms listed on these pages.

Symptoms of a stroke

What is the outlook?

Every year, around 100,000 people in the UK have a stroke. Most recover well, although about 15 percent die within the first three weeks. Most of those who die lose consciousness at the time of the stroke and suffer from severe paralysis for the first three days. The cause of death is normally either a massive cerebral haemorrhage, which accounts for about 80 percent of deaths, damage to a very large number of cells, or a stroke in the brain stem, which controls vital functions such as breathing and heartbeat.

Possible complications

Even when the patient has survived the original stroke, there is still a risk of complications, which could be fatal without treatment. After a stroke, the dead brain cells swell with fluid (cerebral oedema) and, because the bony skull

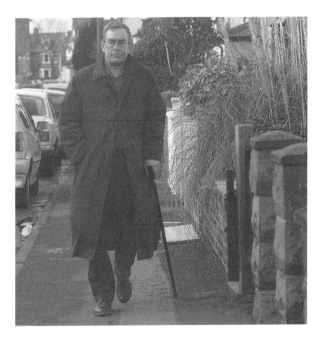

It is common to need a stick for the first few months after a stroke, but many people recover sufficiently to be able to walk unaided.

allows little room for expansion, this puts pressure on nearby, healthy cells, which stop functioning. In the most severe cases, the person loses consciousness and will die without treatment. In less serious strokes—the majority of cases—the fluid is re-absorbed over a period of about three months. This re-absorption is most rapid in the first two to three weeks, which is why stroke patients often experience such a rapid improvement during that time

There is a real risk that an elderly, semi-conscious person will contract a chest infection (see p. 27), so they will need regular chest physiotherapy (see p. 30) to prevent this. A person who is bed-ridden and immobile is also at risk of developing a thrombus in a vein (deep vein thrombosis). Wearing support stockings and taking anticoagulant drugs (see p. 28) can help to prevent this. If an embolus breaks off it may block an artery in the lungs (a pulmonary embolism), which is potentially fatal.

Even though most people do not have a second stroke, the risk at this time is higher than in someone who has never had a stroke. The patient is also at risk of a heart attack at this time—the causes of stroke are so similar to those of heart disease (see p. 12) that heart attacks are the commonest cause of death in stroke patients.

The recovery period

Few people recover fully from a major stroke, but there is usually an initial spurt of recovery during the first three months, and continuing, more gradual recovery for a year or longer. Fluid is re-absorbed, relieving pressure on brain cells, new nerve pathways develop, other brain cells assume the functions of the dead ones and the patient makes a number of adaptations to compensate for any remaining disability.

YOU REALLY NEED TO KNOW

◆ The most critical period for the patient is the first three weeks after a stroke.

◆ Depending on the severity of the stroke, recovery can take anything from three weeks to over a year.

◆ Full recovery from a stroke is rare, but many patients show considerable improvement in both their physical and mental capabilities.

What is the outlook?

What else could it be?

✓ Some people may have an epileptic fit during a stroke.

✗ Vertigo (a feeling of spinning) without any other symptoms is very rarely due to stroke.

If there is any suspicion that someone has suffered a stroke, however minor the symptoms, always seek medical advice. A number of other conditions can cause symptoms similar to those of a stroke.

Alzheimer's disease

The most common cause of dementia, Alzheimer's disease is an incurable degenerative disorder of the brain. The first symptom is usually a failing memory, followed by difficulties with speech that progress to a disabling confusion.

Unlike a stroke, the condition is not caused by a disruption in the blood supply to the brain, but its symptoms are similar to those caused by multiple infarcts (see p. 14), which can often be prevented or treated effectively. Never take it for granted that a failing memory in an elderly relative is the result of Alzheimer's or the dementia of old age—always check with the individual's doctor.

Brain tumour

A brain tumour—whether harmless or not—can cause symptoms that are very similar to those of a stroke and, like a stroke, can start very suddenly. Symptoms that develop after a tumour has been removed may be put down to a secondary tumour when, in fact, a stroke is responsible. Again, it is vital to check with the individual's doctor without delay.

Multiple sclerosis

The symptoms of multiple sclerosis, which affects the brain and spinal cord, include temporary paralysis, double vision and tremors. Multiple sclerosis affects twice as many women as men and usually becomes apparent under the age of 40, but its symptoms can sometimes be confused with those of a stroke.

Epilepsy

An epileptic fit (an abnormal and rapid firing of nerve cells in the cortex of the brain) can be mistaken for a stroke. A severe epileptic fit can leave a person suffering temporary paralysis from a few hours to a few days.

Head injury

A blow to the head can cause swelling in the brain, which can mimic a stroke caused by a haemorrhage. Even if there is no swelling, the sudden jarring of the brain against the bony skull can cause the brain cells to become overexcited and fire off unusual and unwanted messages similar to those of epilepsy.

GET EXPERT ADVICE

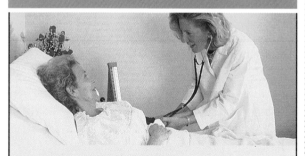

Anyone who exhibits the symptoms of a stroke—however mild—should be examined by a doctor to rule out the possibility of a number of other conditions and decide on the most appropriate treatment.

1

YOU REALLY NEED TO KNOW

◆ The symptoms of a number of conditions are very similar to those of a stroke, so do not simply assume that someone has had a stroke—always seek medical advice.

◆ A CT brain scan can be very helpful in identifying other causes of stroke-like symptoms.

◆ CT scans done within a few hours of a stroke may be normal even in people who have had very large strokes. Small strokes may never show on the scan.

What else could it be?

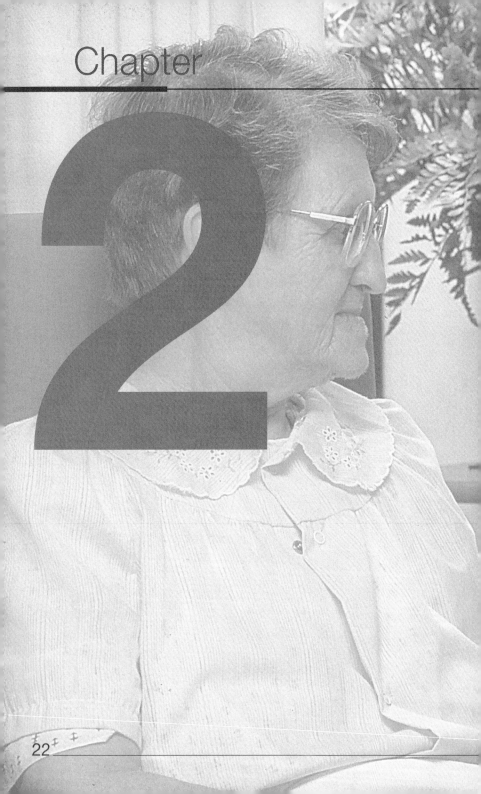

Chapter

2

DIAGNOSIS &
TREATMENT

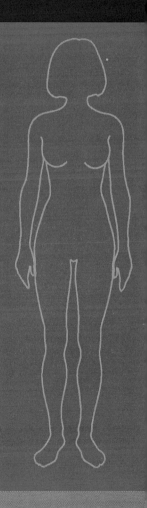

Tests and assessments

✓ Emergency surgery helps some five percent of stroke patients.

✓ Emergency surgery can be particularly helpful after either a subarachnoid haemorrhage or brain haemorrhage, to relieve pressure.

People who have had strokes are usually cared for in hospital at first, either in a general medical ward or a specialized stroke unit. When the patient arrives, the medical staff will take a full family and medical history, either from the patient, if he or she is conscious, a relative or the family doctor. In the early stages it is hard to pin down what type of stroke has occurred, so the doctor will carry out a range of tests to diagnose this and eliminate other problems.

Tests after a stroke

A number of tests may be carried out after a stroke. These include:

◆ Blood tests to check for diabetes, anaemia and sickle cell disease.

◆ Chest X-ray to see if the heart is enlarged (a sign of high blood pressure).

◆ CT (computerized tomography) scan. A CT scanner is similar to an X-ray machine but takes horizontal

THE ROAD TO RECOVERY

It is extremely difficult to give an accurate idea of how recovery may proceed after a stroke. Some severely affected patients make a good recovery, while others who seem less affected by the stroke itself may not improve as much. Generally, stroke patients tend to recover their abilities in the sequence given below, and most achieve reasonable independence within a year.

◆ Regain consciousness

◆ Regain control of bladder and bowels

pictures in thin slices through the brain. These reveal any haemorrhage or tumour, but cannot show an area of dead tissue in the first few hours.

◆ MRI (magnetic resonance imaging) scan. Like a CT scan, this reveals a haemorrhage or tumour and can also show damaged tissue very quickly.

◆ ECG (electrocardiogram) to check for heart disease or signs of a recent heart attack.

◆ Carotid ultrasound to check that the arteries in the neck that supply the brain are not furred up.

Assessment after a stroke

The doctor will give the patient a full physical examination to pinpoint the area of the brain that has been affected and the extent of any damage. Questions that need to be answered include: Is there any paralysis of the limbs or face? Which side of the body is affected? Is there any loss of sensation? Is there any alteration in vision? Is there any confusion? (see p. 16).

◆ Sit upright in a chair
◆ Swallow correctly and feed themselves
◆ Carry out basic personal care, such as cleaning teeth, washing face, brushing hair and so on
◆ Walk with help
◆ Move from bed to chair and back again safely
◆ Walk independently with a stick or a tripod
◆ Dress (shoelaces and buttons may still be a problem)
◆ Cope safely with stairs and a bath

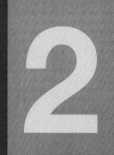

YOU REALLY NEED TO KNOW

◆ Two-thirds of people who cannot walk independently during the first few days after a stroke do so within a year.

◆ Some 90 percent of stroke patients regain the ability to feed themselves.

◆ The symptom least likely to disappear is paralysis in an arm, particularly when the paralysis has lasted for more than three months.

Tests and assessments

25

Hospital treatment

Usually a stroke patient will stay in hospital for anything from a couple of days to a few months, although in some cases home care is given right from the start. Elderly patients are likely to stay in hospital for longer.

After the initial tests, assessment and diagnosis, the medical team starts to develop a care and rehabilitation plan. The physiotherapist (see p. 30), occupational therapist (see p. 32) and speech therapist (see p. 34) make their assessments, while the doctors and nurses act to prevent a further stroke (see p. 28) and deal with any secondary complications. A dietician may suggest dietary changes to reduce high blood pressure.

Monitoring and routine

All stroke patients are monitored at regular, frequent intervals for at least the first 48 hours, checking the level of consciousness, blood pressure, and mental and physical state. Much of the hospital routine is concerned with ensuring a patient's safety and guarding against other complications. If the patient has swallowing difficulties and there is a risk of choking, he may be fed through a tube for the first few days. A catheter to drain urine from the bladder may also be needed.

Secondary complications

Possible complications the team will be on the look-out for include:

◆ Pressure sores—paralysis may mean the patient cannot move even when lying for too long in the same position, especially if sensation has been affected.

◆ Dehydration—problems with swallowing may make it difficult for the patient to drink fluids so he may need a drip to keep fluid levels up.

◆ Chest infection—swallowing problems may cause food, drink or saliva to go into the patient's lungs instead of being swallowed. Mucus may also build up. Physiotherapy can help.

◆ Deep vein thrombosis or pulmonary embolus—lying immobile means that blood circulates more slowly in the leg veins. If the flow is slow enough, the blood may clot (thrombosis). If part of the clot breaks off, becoming an embolus, it may lodge in the lungs (pulmonary embolism).

Starting rehabilitation

Although stroke patients tire easily, they shouldn't remain inactive—short bursts of activity separated by long periods of rest are best in the early days. The sooner patients can sit up and start doing things for themselves the better. Even small advances help morale.

YOU REALLY NEED TO KNOW

◆ During the first few days in hospital, staff will put together a care and rehabilitation plan. This involves physiotherapy, occupational therapy and speech therapy, as well as medical and nursing care.

◆ While a stroke patient should not overdo things, activity is good for morale and improves rehabilitation.

PREVENTING PRESSURE SORES

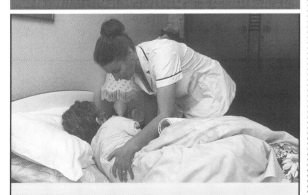

A patient who is paralyzed will find it difficult to move in bed and so is at increased risk of developing pressure sores. Regular turning by nurses helps to prevent them.

Hospital treatment

Hospital treatment

✓ High blood pressure is a major cause of both heart attacks and strokes.

✓ Make arrangements with your doctor to have your blood pressure checked on a regular basis.

When are drugs prescribed?

No drugs currently available can reverse the effects of a stroke, so the main aim of treatment is rehabilitation (see p. 30). Doctors generally only prescribe drugs to reduce the risk of another stroke occurring, and the type of drug depends on the cause of the original stroke. Drugs are never prescribed until the cause has been determined, because if, for example, a stroke patient who had suffered a brain haemorrhage were to be given a drug designed to prevent clot formation, the drug itself would increase the amount of damage caused by the original stroke.

DRUGS TO LOWER BLOOD PRESSURE

Seventy-five percent of stroke patients suffer from long-standing high blood pressure (hypertension). The drugs these patients are given are designed to reduce blood pressure and so reduce the chances of another stroke occurring. They are:

◆ Water tablets (diuretics)—increase the rate at which water and salts are excreted from the kidneys so lessening the tension in the arteries.

◆ Beta-blockers—slow the heart rate and lower the blood pressure by partially blocking the action of the hormones adrenaline and noradrenaline.

◆ Alpha-blockers—work in a similar way to beta-blockers and are often used if the patient also suffers from diabetes or heart failure.

◆ Calcium antagonists—relax the muscles of the arteries so that their walls expand.

What drugs are prescribed?

Two basic types of drug are used: those that lower blood pressure (see chart) and those that prevent the blood clotting. If the medical team is sure that the stroke was caused by a blood clot, the patient may be given drugs to make the blood less sticky and thick and so less likely to form further clots. These drugs do not dissolve an existing clot but they do prevent new ones forming.

Aspirin and alternatives

Aspirin is the most commonly prescribed blood-thinning drug. It is given not only to stroke patients but also to people who have experienced transient ischaemic attacks (see p. 14). The dose required to thin the blood is smaller than that needed when the drug is used as a painkiller, but the patient must take the prescribed amount every day for the rest of his life.

A drug called dipyridamole has recently been shown to double the effect of small doses of aspirin in decreasing the risk of further stroke and is now often used alongside aspirin. Doctors do not yet know whether it is effective by itself. For patients who cannot take aspirin—about one percent of people are allergic to it—another new drug, clopidogrel, can be given.

Two other drugs that reduce the blood's ability to clot are warfarin and heparin. These are especially useful for patients who also suffer from an irregular heartbeat (atrial fibrillation). In this condition, some blood tends to stay in the heart instead of being pumped through the body. As a result, it can become more sticky and likely to clot. Any clots that form may eventually pass through the body and become lodged in the small arteries of the brain, causing a stroke.

YOU REALLY NEED TO KNOW

◆ If you suffer a stroke—or are the friend or relative of someone who has had a stroke—make sure that the hospital doctors are told about any medication taken.

◆ Aspirin reduces the risk of further strokes by a third. Treatment with aspirin should start immediately after a TIA or mini-stroke.

◆ Heparin is usually administered through an intravenous drip and so is generally only given in hospital.

Hospital treatment

Physiotherapy

Physiotherapy can start almost immediately after a stroke, unless it was particularly severe. Even an unconscious or severely disabled, bed-ridden patient may need physiotherapy to keep her lungs clear, and so reduce the risk of getting a chest infection.

Immediately after a stroke, any paralyzed muscles are limp (hypotonic), but their condition changes gradually over the next few days and they become taut (hypertonic, or spastic). While the patient is immobile, there is a risk of developing a deep vein thrombosis in the calf muscles. Wearing support stockings and, sometimes, giving anticoagulant drugs (see p. 28) helps prevent this.

During the muscles' taut stage, the physiotherapist regularly moves the limbs through their natural range of movement in order to reduce spasticity and prevent problems in the joints.

Starting rehabilitation

Because the likely success rate of physiotherapy is good, the physiotherapist's main role is to help get the patient's rehabilitation underway as soon as possible. The precise aim of treatment depends on the severity of the stroke, which parts of the body have been affected, the initial speed of recovery and the patient's lifestyle and rehabilitation goals. Each "goal", such as learning to walk again, is broken down into its component movements, so that each movement can be practised and perfected more easily.

Rehabilitation treatment usually starts in the hospital ward or stroke unit. The patient is given exercises specifically designed to trigger the slightest response or twitch in paralyzed muscles and help reduce spasticity. At first, some patients may find this process difficult, frustrating and tiring, but it is essential to long-term recovery. The physiotherapist also teaches the patient how to balance when sitting and how to move from a bed to a chair and vice versa. Two physiotherapists work together to teach the patient how to stand, how to transfer her weight from one leg to the other and how to take her first few steps.

The next stage

Once recovery is underway, treatment takes place in the specialist physiotherapy department, where it can be more intensive. The patient uses a range of equipment, including parallel bars to practise walking, mats for special exercises and special stools and chairs to practise standing and sitting.

KEEPING UP THE GOOD WORK

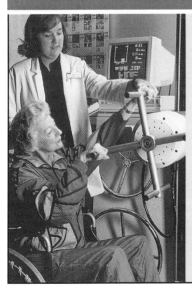

Physiotherapy does not end when the patient leaves hospital, but continues either on an outpatient basis or in her own home. The patient is given an exercise routine, which is also carefully explained to her carer.

◆ Physiotherapy plays a major role in restoring functions damaged by a stroke.

◆ The amount of time spent on physiotherapy each day depends on the hospital routine and how much treatment each individual can take without getting too tired.

Physiotherapy

Occupational therapy

✓ Occupational therapy has evolved over the past 20 years. The emphasis now is on restoring as much independence as possible.

✓ Occupational therapists encourage patients to take up or continue with hobbies and other pastimes.

While physiotherapy concentrates on the correct movement of the limbs and body, occupational therapy (OT) is mainly concerned with helping stroke patients to regain useful practical functions—for example, the ones you need to use cutlery and eat a meal. It aims to help patients maximize their ability to perform everyday tasks, to increase both their independence and their quality of life.

The treatment plan

Once the patient's condition has stabilized, the occupational therapist assesses the degree of damage the stroke has caused and puts together a treatment plan that reflects the patient's priorities and needs. The level of independence that each individual wishes to achieve—and is capable of achieving—varies, and the treatment plan will reflect this. For example, while most elderly people want to recover sufficiently to carry out

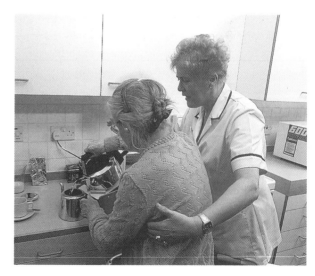

Relearning the skills needed for independent living boosts patients' morale and improves their quality of life.

everyday chores independently, they may not wish to put in all the hard work needed to return to some of their previous activities, such as DIY or embroidery. A younger person, on the other hand, may wish to regain as many of her old skills as possible.

Most stroke patients are given special tasks and activities that help them relearn the movements necessary for tasks such as washing, using the lavatory, eating and dressing. Specialist aids are available to help with this—for example, special cutlery to make it easier to cut up food and move it from plate to mouth. The occupational therapist will also try to minimize any emotional or psychological problems by involving the patient in various hobbies and pastimes and making her feel that she still has plenty to contribute, both to her family and to the wider community.

Mind games

As well as causing a range of physical disabilities, a stroke can affect the way the brain perceives and interprets information and uses it to make decisions. Emotional stability, concentration and memory can also be affected. For example, a patient may be unaware of objects placed to the side of her body affected by the stroke, be unable to understand numbers (and therefore manage money or the telephone), have a short attention span or find distances difficult to judge.

The occupational therapist assesses any such problems and uses various techniques to stimulate the brain to relearn the appropriate responses. Often these appear at first sight to be fairly simple games, such as bingo, but they are in fact carefully thought out to help the patient's recovery.

YOU REALLY NEED TO KNOW

◆ The main aim of occupational therapy is to restore the more sophisticated movements necessary for everyday tasks and, where appropriate, to restore brain functions concerned with understanding and thought.

◆ Occupational therapists can provide a wide range of specialist aids that help with everyday chores, and prepare the home for the special needs of a stroke patient.

Occupational therapy

Speech therapy

STROKE FACTS

Many people who experience difficulties with language immediately after a stroke improve dramatically in the first few weeks.

About a third of all stroke patients have difficulty swallowing (dysphagia) in the first few days. Speech therapists can help, because swallowing and voice production use many of the same muscles.

During the first few days and weeks following a stroke, nearly half of all stroke patients have problems with speech, reading or writing. Some have difficulty in recognizing words or understanding their meaning. Communication problems are more common when the right side of the body is affected, because the main language control centres are in the left cerebral hemisphere of the brain (see p. 14).

Types of communication problem

Speech therapists classify communication difficulties in a number of ways. In expressive or motor dysphasia, patients can understand the spoken and written word, but cannot use the correct words to express themselves in speech or writing. This varies in severity: some patients cannot form any words; others speak fluently but the words come out as meaningless phrases. Sometimes the word used may be close to the one wanted, but at other times there is no similarity between them.

In receptive or sensory dysphasia, patients have difficulty understanding spoken or written words, while in dysarthria, speech may be slurred or weak due to paralysis or weakness of the muscles in the face, tongue and throat that control speech.

Communication problems mainly affect people who have had a stroke in the right side of the brain, affecting the left side of their body. This type of stroke does not normally result in any language problems (unless the patient is one of the few left-handed people whose language centre is in the right side of their brain), but damage to centres in the right side can affect how an individual interprets and uses language. For example, he may lose his sense of humour, along with the knowledge

TALKING IT OVER

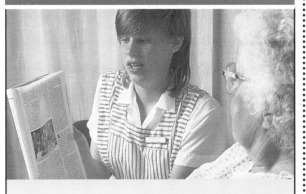

Speech therapy often continues over a period of time, and the therapist needs to explain any problems to the rest of the rehabilitation team and the family so that they know the best way of communicating with the patient.

of social niceties, such as taking turns to talk and listening when another person is talking, and he may speak in a deadpan manner, with no accompanying facial expressions or gestures.

The treatment plan

The speech therapist assesses the patient's condition and draws up an individual treatment plan. This will usually involve teaching the patient the language skills he has lost, using similar techniques to those used to teach children to talk, read and write. For example, the therapist may use flash cards to identify common objects, and may use repeated vowel sounds and other elements of speech to re-educate the patient's muscles and help him relearn old habits.

2

YOU REALLY NEED TO KNOW

◆ Around half of all stroke patients have communication problems during the first two weeks. Speech therapists classify these in a variety of ways.

◆ The speech therapist draws up an individual treatment plan for each patient, according to the type of communication problem involved.

◆ The general confusion experienced by around a third of all stroke patients, especially the elderly, is not classed as a communication problem in itself, but as a sign of general brain dysfunction.

Speech therapy

Chapter

3

COPING AT HOME

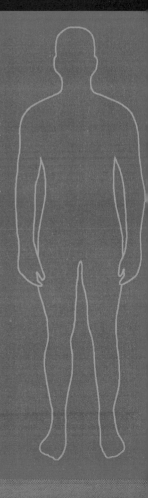

Before going home

A stroke patient's capabilities are assessed before she leaves hospital. An occupational therapist and a social worker also carry out a home assessment to find out what aids or alterations are needed to help the patient and carer to cope. They look at the layout—for example, if the bedroom and bathroom are on the same floor—and whether any adaptations are needed to make life easier for the patient and her carer. Sometimes the stroke patient goes home for a few days in order for the assessment to be carried out.

HOW A HOME ASSESSMENT IS DONE

A home assessment will look at the following questions regarding a patient's capabilities, her home and exactly what her carer can do.

THE PATIENT

◆ Can the patient live independently without any help from social services?

◆ Can she climb stairs and take a bath in safety?

◆ Can she live alone or with a partner?

◆ Are there other family members or friends who can help?

◆ How mobile is the patient and how near are the local shops?

THE HOME

◆ Is the front door wide enough to take a wheelchair and is there an outside step?

◆ If the patient cannot manage stairs, is there a downstairs lavatory or will she need a commode?

◆ Is there room for a bed downstairs?

◆ Do chairs and bed need raising for safety and ease of use?

Advance planning

The occupational therapist and social worker arrange for any alterations and aids to be in place before the patient comes home for good. This can range from moving the bathroom to the ground floor to supplying hoists for bathing, safety handles and bars in the bathroom, long-handled taps, which are easier to turn on and off, non-slip mats to hold cups and plates in place, specially designed cutlery and china and a raised or lowered bed to make getting in and out safer and easier.

◆ Can kitchen appliances be reached easily or do the surfaces need to be lowered?

◆ Are door handles and locks easy to use?

◆ Is the floor suitable for a wheelchair, sticks or a tripod?

◆ Are rails and other aids needed in the lavatory and bathroom and on the stairs?

THE CARER

◆ Is the carer the main wage earner and will daytime cover be needed?

◆ If the patient was the main wage earner, how will the carer and patient cope financially?

◆ Is the carer sufficiently robust to take on full-time care, or will outside help, for example from community nurses, be needed?

◆ Does the carer need any training from the community physiotherapist to enable him to cope with the physical demands of moving the victim around?

YOU REALLY NEED TO KNOW

◆ An occupational therapist and a social worker will make an assessment of the patient's capabilities and what facilities are available at home before she leaves hospital.

◆ Specialist aids will be provided and changes made to the home if necessary.

◆ The carer's abilities will also be assessed and any necessary extra help or training provided.

◆ Driving will probably not be possible until recovery is complete, and may not be advisable then. Always check with your doctor.

Before going home

Helping with mobility

Physiotherapists teach stroke patients the correct ways to lie, sit and stand while they are in hospital. Once at home, though, it is easy to slip into bad habits, especially if there has not been enough time to teach carers the correct positions for the patient.

Time spent in bed

It is important for a stroke patient to spend as little time as possible in bed. However, when there is a degree of paralysis, it is important that he can move around the bed safely and change position, not just for comfort but to reduce the risk of pressure sores or a deep vein thrombosis (see p. 18).

The patient needs good support when sitting in bed, so place firm pillows against a solid headrest. Many stroke patients tend to slump over toward the affected

---

SLEEPING COMFORTABLY

If the patient is suffering from paralysis, the best sleeping position depends on whether he is lying on the affected or unaffected side. Paralyzed limbs must be supported at all times.

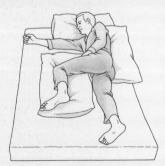

LYING ON THE AFFECTED SIDE

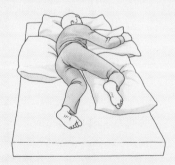

LYING ON THE UNAFFECTED SIDE

TURNING OVER IN BED

Everyone changes their position during sleep, but those with paralysis are often unable to do this. As a result, a stroke patient may need to be turned every few hours during the night—carers should ask for outside help. If you ever have to turn the patient on your own, follow these instructions.

◆ Turn the patient's head in the direction in which you want his body to roll.

◆ Bend his top arm and leg and bring the arm forward over his chest and the leg over his lower thigh.

◆ If his top arm is strong enough, he should be able to pull himself over, perhaps using a rope or sheet tied to the side of the bed to help. If he is not strong enough, you may have to turn him yourself.

side, especially in the early weeks, and may need extra pillows to help them stay upright. Rest a paralyzed or weak arm on a pillow to make sure the shoulder joint is not stretched, as it can easily be damaged.

A monkey pole with a triangular hand grip can be fitted at the head of the bed to help the patient move up the bed when he wants to sit up or get out of bed. The carer stands on the patient's weak side, facing the head of the bed, and bends the patient's legs, so that his feet are flat on the mattress. The paralyzed or weak arm is then placed over the carer's shoulder and the patient pushes up with his legs and pulls up on the monkey pole. The carer supports the weak side and prevents the patient from overbalancing.

Helping with mobility

Helping with mobility

✓ At first, some stroke patients need help to walk safely. But by six months, over 80 percent can walk unaided around the house and for short distances outside.

✓ There is a much greater chance of recovering full use of a paralyzed leg than a paralyzed arm.

Getting out of bed

It is vital to encourage a stroke patient to get up and about as soon as he possibly can. But first, the patient must learn how to get out of bed safely, regain his balance and relearn the basic techniques of walking. This may be a very slow process, but it is essential that you both persevere.

Place a chair or the wheelchair, if the patient is using one, next to the bed. It should be parallel to the bed and on the unaffected side of his body. Ideally, the mattress should be at a height that allows the patient's feet to be placed comfortably flat on the ground when he is sitting on the bed, and the seat of the chair should be at the same height. Help the patient to lie on his unaffected

MOVING FROM BED TO CHAIR

Once the patient is seated on the edge of the bed, stand in front of him with your arms around his back and your feet and knees in front of his affected leg, to prevent the weak knee from buckling. Help him stand, encouraging him to place his weight on both legs, then turn him round to sit down slowly in the chair, bending at the waist rather than falling backward.

side (see p. 40), and ask him to push up with his good arm while you swing his legs over the edge of the bed. Take great care to support the patient's affected side while you do this, and make sure he doesn't overbalance. Then help him to stand, following the procedure described in the box opposite, and finally turn him round to sit in the chair or wheelchair.

Preparing to walk

A patient who is still unable to walk on leaving hospital will be given physiotherapy, either at home or in hospital as an outpatient. Treatment aims to revitalize muscles and make walking possible again, using assisted exercises, some of them with the help of parallel bars. It is important that carers try to be present during the physiotherapy sessions so that they can learn the correct way to help the patient and encourage him to practise the exercises properly at home.

The first stage of relearning how to walk involves acquiring the ability to balance and to stand confidently for several minutes. If the patient's leg is severely paralyzed, it may need two people—one of them a physiotherapist or nurse—to help with this. Otherwise, the carer must stand on the weak side of the patient's body and support it if necessary.

The next step is for the patient to learn how to transfer his weight from one leg to the other. To help him do this, stand facing his affected side with one foot in front of his weak leg and the other behind it. Place one arm behind the patient's back with the other supporting his weak arm. If his arm is paralyzed, you should place it over your shoulder, but be careful not to pull on the patient's shoulder joint.

YOU REALLY NEED TO KNOW

◆ When a stroke causes weakening or paralysis of the leg, the first steps toward regaining the ability to walk involve learning how to balance and how to transfer weight from one foot to the other.

◆ The length of time it takes to achieve this varies from person to person, according to the severity of the damage caused by the stroke. Essential to the process are repetition and perseverance, as well as the help of a carer.

Helping with mobility

Helping with mobility

First steps

Once the patient can put weight on the affected limb and can balance, walking—with help—becomes possible. When he finally takes his first few unaided steps, it will give his confidence a huge boost, reassuring him that he will eventually regain his independence.

It is important to prepare the patient's home beforehand. Position comfortable chairs in strategic sites so the patient can walk from one to another. Move any objects that might be in the way. Place solid pieces of furniture where they can be used as extra support, and remove any rugs or mats that might cause a slip.

The physiotherapist will make sure the patient has a tripod or stick of the correct height, which he should hold in his good hand. If the patient's knee is not strong

WALKING WITH SUPPORT

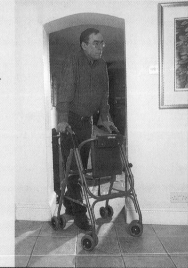

Once the patient can take a few steps, regular practice—with ever-reducing help— often brings about remarkable improvements. A wheeled tripod, like the one shown, is often easier to use than one that has to be lifted.

enough to avoid buckling, make sure he wears a temporary knee brace.

When the patient is ready to walk, stand facing his weak side. Put one arm around his back and support his weak arm with the other (or place this arm over your shoulder). Ask him to put his weight on his good leg and then take a step forward with the affected one, moving the tripod forward at the same time. Then ask him to transfer his weight on to the affected leg, carrying some of the weight on the tripod. You may have to place your front leg in front of his affected leg to give extra support. Make sure that he keeps his balance throughout the entire step before he attempts the next one.

Climbing stairs

The last hurdle to overcome is learning to climb up and down stairs without help. Stroke patients should not try to do this until they can walk confidently with only minimal assistance. Again, thorough preparations are essential. If there is no handrail on the stairs, ask your social worker or occupational therapist to arrange for one to be fitted.

When climbing the stairs, the patient should grasp the handrail with his good hand and move his good leg up to the next step. You should stand directly behind him, holding the rail with one hand and placing your other hand at his waist on his weak side. The patient then lifts his weak leg up on to the same step—you may have to help bend his knee up and forward. Encourage him to rest on the step until he has regained his balance.

To come down the stairs, the patient should lead with his affected leg, and you should stand in front of him, on the next step down. Again, take one step at a time.

YOU REALLY NEED TO KNOW

◆ Repetition and patience are the keywords when it comes to learning how to walk again.

◆ Mastering the first few steps can be a considerable morale booster.

Helping with mobility

Coping around the home

Talk to your doctor and occupational therapist about exactly what is needed before making expensive alterations to your home.

In the bedroom

◆ A single bed is better than a double because it gives the carer easy access to the patient's right and left sides.

◆ Choose a firm, but not too firm, mattress—this makes it easier for the patient to move around in bed, and to get in and out.

◆ Tie a rope ladder to the head of the bed. The patient can grab hold of it to help move around. Alternatively, you can fit a monkey pole (see p.41) at the head of the bed.

◆ Make sure that clothes are easy to put on—doing up buttons one-handed is nearly impossible. You can buy special button hooks to help.

◆ The patient should not wear slippers—they do not give enough support to a paralyzed or weak ankle.

◆ Allow plenty of time for dressing and discreetly check the results—some patients forget how to dress ("dressing dyspraxia") and put their clothes on back to front, wear their shoes on the wrong feet and so on.

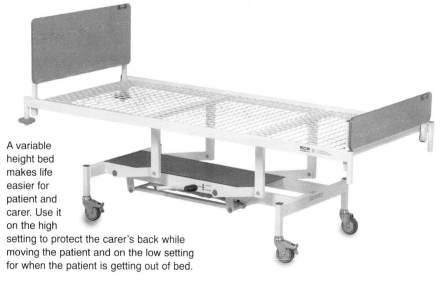

A variable height bed makes life easier for patient and carer. Use it on the high setting to protect the carer's back while moving the patient and on the low setting for when the patient is getting out of bed.

In the bathroom and toilet

◆ Ask your occupational therapist about aids, such as non-slip bath mats and transfer boards.

◆ If you are not strong enough to help the patient with bathing, ask for a community nurse to assist you. Using a plastic chair under a shower may be easier.

◆ At first, some patients may need help with personal grooming—such as shaving or putting on make-up. Take the time to do this properly, as knowing you look good has a positive impact on morale.

◆ Independence and privacy in the toilet are vitally important to most people. Ask your occupational therapist or social worker about aids, such as a raised toilet seat and support bars.

◆ Have a commode on hand if the patient has difficulty getting up and down the stairs to reach the toilet.

In the kitchen

◆ If the patient is using a wheelchair, place a few everyday items, such as a kettle, mug, tea and coffee, on a table at the correct height.

◆ Ask the occupational therapist about specialist aids, such as non-slip plates and mats, one-handed cutlery and a stand to make using the kettle safer.

◆ Make sure the kitchen floor is kept dry (to avoid slips).

In the sitting room

◆ Check that the patient's chair is comfortable. It should have a padded back that is high enough to support the neck and wide arms.

◆ Make sure there is a telephone near the patient's chair so she can call for help when alone—ask your social worker about installing a careline or buy a mobile.

**YOU REALLY
NEED TO KNOW**

◆ Social services give grants to adapt homes for use by stroke patients as well as supplying specialist aids. Ask the social worker or occupational therapist for details.

◆ Respect your own physical limits and do not try to do anything that is beyond you.

Coping around the home

Coping around the home

Regaining independence

Rehabilitation can be a slow, painstaking process for patient and carer. It is natural for a carer to try to reduce the patient's frustrations and lessen her difficulties by helping too much, but doing so is counterproductive. Indeed, it is vital that you encourage the patient to do as

REHABILITATION DOS AND DON'TS

DO...

◆ Break tasks down into small, achievable components and try not to rush things. Bear in mind the advice "little and often".

◆ Use two bedside tables: put a bell (to call for help), a light, radio and other essentials on the unaffected side, but place something, such as a book, on the affected side to encourage the patient to use her weak arm.

◆ Stay patient and calm—stroke patients often feel angry and frustrated at their inability to perform simple tasks and sometimes take their feelings out on their carer.

◆ Encourage the patient and praise any small signs of improvement and progress, while reminding her of any improvements she has already made.

◆ Encourage a stroke patient to keep herself smart and well-groomed.

◆ Explain to family and friends what the problems are: because a stroke patient may not be able to talk sense does not necessarily mean that she cannot understand just as well as she did before the stroke. Talking to her as you would to a small child only increases any sense of depression and frustration she may be feeling.

much as possible without help, even though she will need assistance with many things in the early days. There are two reasons for this: first, regaining independence raises morale and increases self-esteem; and second, it is only as a result of trying and trying again that the patient will realize just how much improvement is possible.

◆ Encourage the patient to continue with any exercises suggested by the medical team, even if they do not seem to be having much effect—recovery does take time and some improvements can be almost imperceptible in the early days.

◆ Bolster the patient's sense of usefulness by asking her to take on any household chores that are within her current capability.

DON'T...

◆ Help with dressing for the sake of speed if the patient can manage to dress on her own—it does not matter how long the process takes.

◆ Help with feeding, even if the result is a mess at first— use a large towel to keep food off the patient's clothes.

◆ Place everything on the patient's "good" side—it is more helpful for a patient with a partially paralyzed arm to use a beaker cup on her weak side than to use a normal cup on her strong side.

◆ Be over-optimistic about the speed of recovery— improvements tend to be small and come gradually, and a stroke patient tires easily.

YOU REALLY NEED TO KNOW

◆ Rehabilitation is more likely to succeed if you let a stroke patient try and achieve tasks for herself.

◆ Don't let the patient become too reliant on others. Encourage all attempts to use the affected limbs as much as possible.

Coping around the home

Diet and lifestyle

There is no reason why a stroke patient should not enjoy most of the same food as anyone else. But stroke patients do have some special problems, which must be taken into account when planning their diet, and changes to diet and lifestyle can do much to help to reduce the risk of suffering a second stroke.

Beneficial changes

The main indirect causes of stroke include high blood pressure, diabetes, high cholesterol and smoking. Patients with diabetes will have their own dietary requirements, which are compatible with a healthy diet for stroke patients, and high blood pressure will probably be treated with drugs. Nevertheless, there are a number of things that a stroke patient can do to help lower his blood pressure and reduce the chances of another stroke.

There is some debate about whether too much salt in the diet increases blood pressure to dangerous levels. However, there is no question that a low-salt diet helps to reduce high blood pressure. There is also evidence that a diet with plenty of fruit and vegetables—aim for five portions a day—protects against a stroke.

Smoking more than doubles the risk of a stroke. A stroke patient who smokes should give up immediately. There is no need to give up alcohol, however. A daily glass or two of wine, say, is thought to reduce the risk of a stroke. But drinking more than this is likely to increase the risk. Ask your family doctor for advice—in particular check whether it is safe to drink alcohol while taking any prescribed medication.

Being very overweight increases blood pressure, and losing weight reduces it. In addition, being overweight makes movement more difficult and so makes rehabilitation slower and more challenging. Ask your doctor about a planned weight-reduction programme and consult the patient's physiotherapist about how he can become more active if necessary.

Watch out for false teeth

False teeth can cause problems, because weakened facial muscles may not be up to the job of keeping them in place. Usually the problem resolves itself as the patient recovers—otherwise he may need to see the dentist to have a new set of dentures fitted.

KEEP HEALTHY WITH FIBRE

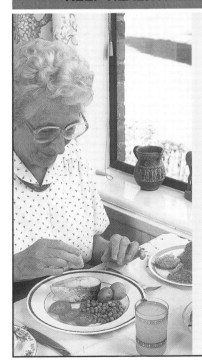

Constipation can be a problem, partly because the patient is not moving about much. Rather than giving laxatives, make sure she eats a high-fibre diet, with plenty of wholemeal bread, brown rice, fruit, vegetables and high-fibre cereals. She should also drink plenty of plain water.

YOU REALLY NEED TO KNOW

◆ A low-salt, low-fat diet that includes plenty of fruit and vegetables can reduce the risk of a stroke occurring.

◆ Smoking doubles the risk of a stroke.

◆ Heavy drinking increases the risk of a stroke; a limited intake of alcohol may reduce it.

◆ Obesity makes a stroke more likely and hampers rehabilitation.

Diet and lifestyle

Diet and lifestyle

Some stroke patients feel embarrassed about their physical and emotional problems and refuse to leave home.

It is important that carers encourage patients to get out and about as much as possible to help with their rehabilitation.

Friends and relatives

Many stroke patients find it difficult to come to terms with changes in their abilities and personal appearance —they may feel a sense of shame and an unwillingness to be seen by others. But humans are social animals and contact with others is important for psychological health. Interests and activities are also vital for morale.

The sooner a stroke patient starts to socialize, the faster he will start to come to terms with the effects of the stroke. Encourage friends and relatives to visit as soon as possible, and make sure the patient does not become a hermit. Cajole him into activity—even though you may have to overcome his feelings of frustration or anger at what he can no longer do.

It can be difficult to persuade friends and relatives to visit a stroke patient. Some people are embarrassed by the physical or mental effects of a stroke and do not

As soon as the patient is sufficiently mobile, encourage him to take up hobbies again. If he enjoys gardening, long-handled tools may make it easier as the gardener does not need to stretch outside a comfortable range of movement.

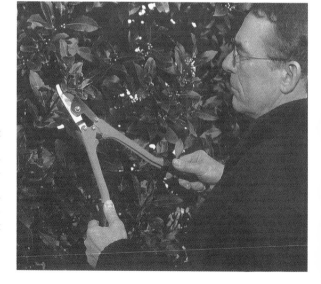

know how to cope—the best solution is to explain exactly what has happened, stressing the chances of recovery. Others may stop visiting because they no longer have any mutual interests. The answer is for you and the patient to make new friends. Join your local stroke club (see p. 78), where you will find people who understand your problems and concerns.

Interests and activities

As well as improving morale, interests and activities provide mental and physical stimulation, both of which are vital to rehabilitation. Some favourite activities may no longer be possible, but new ones can be substituted—ask the occupational therapist (see p. 32) for suggestions. In some cases, a patient's determination to recover sufficiently to enjoy a favourite activity can be a major spur to rehabilitation.

You can also try the following ideas:

◆ When the patient is fit enough both physically and mentally, encourage him to go out unaccompanied—to the shops, for example, or to meet a friend.

◆ Encourage hobbies, such as reading or chess.

◆ If the patient is keen on sport but can't yet travel to watch it live, invite friends round to watch it on television.

◆ Make a positive effort to take up any activities you can enjoy doing together, such as playing cards, doing the crossword, reading to each other or doing a jigsaw.

◆ Encourage daily light exercise—depending on the patient's level of recovery. Walking, swimming and games such as bowls are all good forms of exercise.

◆ If necessary, ask about games and facilities available for wheelchair-bound stroke patients at your local leisure centre or disabled club.

YOU REALLY NEED TO KNOW

◆ Seeing friends and relatives and indulging in interests and activities not only improves morale but also provides the mental and physical stimulation that is essential for recovery.

◆ The occupational therapist should be able to suggest a number of activities that the patient will be able to manage.

Diet and lifestyle

53

Possible problems

People often claim that an individual's personality has changed after a stroke, but major personality changes are very rare.

A stroke can lessen a person's control over characteristics that were always present. An individual who previously bottled up anger, for example, may now display it with little provocation.

Individuals vary in their emotional and psychological reactions to what has happened to them. In general, they tend to be, by turns, anxious, frustrated, angry and depressed. It is important for a carer to appreciate these problems, talking them through with the family doctor and occupational therapist, if necessary. The patient can then be reassured that such problems are a normal part of having a stroke and not a sign of mental illness. In rare cases, however, the patient's confusion persists beyond what is to be expected in the first few days (see p. 16).

Anxiety, frustration and anger

The sudden shock of a stroke turns life upside down for most patients. The future seems uncertain, and anxiety about the chances of recovery is usually acute. In many cases, this feeling persists for several weeks and may deepen into depression if recovery turns out to be slower than expected.

TALK THINGS OVER WITH YOUR DOCTOR

It is important for carers to appreciate that a patient may have emotional and psychological problems in the months following a stroke. Anxiety, frustration, anger and depression are common. Talking it through with the doctor can help you to understand the problems.

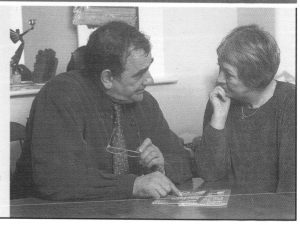

Frustration, irritability and anger are common, too, as patients find themselves unable to carry out everyday tasks they used to take for granted. Emotional outbursts are to be expected: for example, difficulties in communication may lead to tears of anger or the good fist being thumped on a table. Such outbursts can be wearing for both patient and carer. Remember, though, that while they appear to be aimed toward others, they are rooted in the patient's own inabilities and frustrations.

Depression

Around 40 percent of stroke patients suffer from depression in the first few months. This can be successfully treated with antidepressants. The severity of the depression varies according to the patient's social and family situation and whether there is any previous history of depression. However, you should always look out for depression and consult your family doctor if you feel that the stroke patient lacks motivation and is behaving in an unco-operative manner.

Two particular danger points can trigger depression during the recovery period. The first follows the recovery "spurt" (see p. 18) that happens in the first three months. The patient may be over-optimistic that recovery will continue at the same pace. Explain that although recovery becomes more gradual, it will still be possible to lead a relatively normal life in the long run.

The second danger point is when the rehabilitation team decides that it has no further part to play in recovery. The patient can sometimes feel abandoned. Reassure her that by continuing with her exercises and working on how to modify the way she carries out tasks, her improvement will continue after therapy has ended.

YOU REALLY NEED TO KNOW

◆ Psychological problems after a stroke are not usually the result of mental illness but of the patient's difficulty in coming to terms with her disabilities and her worries about the chances and progress of recovery.

◆ Consult the family doctor if you suspect a stroke victim is suffering from depression. Lack of motivation and co-operation may both be indicators of depression.

Possible problems

Possible problems

Central post-stroke pain affects only two percent of all stroke patients. The problem can develop at any time during the first two years of recovery and rehabilitation.

Central post-stroke pain is most common in people under 50.

Post-stroke pain

Pain is not normally a direct effect of a stroke (see p.16), as brain tissue has no pain receptors. But if the brain swells as the result of a haemorrhage, pressure on the skull, which does contain pain receptors, can cause a severe headache. This is normally relieved by treatment in the days immediately following the stroke.

Pain can be a problem during recovery and rehabilitation. The most common type is joint and muscle pain, as a result of limited movement following paralysis, or poor handling when moving the patient. More rarely, there is a nagging pain in one or more parts of the body which cannot be relieved, known as "central post-stroke pain".

Frozen shoulder

"Frozen shoulder", also known as adhesive capsulitis, is the most common post-stroke joint and muscle pain. It is an inflammation of the fibrous capsule of the shoulder

WAYS TO RELIEVE PAIN

Antidepressants can be used to reduce spinal cord activity. A drug called mexiletine is also sometimes prescribed. If the pain persists, the doctor may recommend implanting an electrical device that relieves pain by stimulating areas of brain tissue or the spine (right).

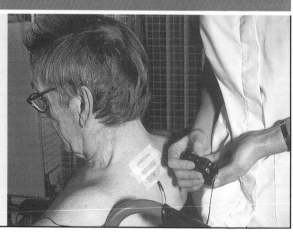

joint, resulting from tiny strains to the short muscles that surround the joint. It severely restricts movement of the joint, causes pain in the upper arm, often with shooting pains down it, and leads to further muscular problems as other muscles, such as those attached to the shoulder blade, are used to compensate.

The risk of a frozen shoulder can be reduced if the patient is moved regularly—every two hours during the early stages of recovery—during the day and night (see p. 41), and by making sure the handling techniques taught by the physiotherapist (see p. 30) are used at all times. If it remains a problem, hydrocortisone injections and physiotherapy may be needed.

Central post-stroke pain

Affecting around two percent of all stroke patients, central post-stroke pain can develop at any time up to about two years after the stroke, and is more common in people under the age of 50.

The pain may affect up to half the body, or only a small part, and may be described as burning, shooting or throbbing. The patient may also lose some or all feeling in the affected area, especially the ability to determine temperature, which can make it difficult to test bath water, for example. If this is a problem, make sure you test the temperature of the water before the patient gets into the bath.

This type of pain is not relieved by even the strongest of painkillers, but a variety of different treatments can be used successfully (see left), depending on the precise nature of the pain. It important to seek medical advice as soon as the problem becomes apparent as the sooner treatment is started, the better.

YOU REALLY NEED TO KNOW

◆ It is important that the stroke patient's position is changed regularly and that all carers use correct handling techniques to guard against muscle and joint pains, such as those experienced with a frozen shoulder.

◆ Central post-stroke pain does not respond to conventional painkillers, but other treatments are available, so seek medical advice if you suspect that it may be a problem.

Possible problems

Possible problems

Do make an effort to keep communicating with the patient and encourage her to respond to you.

Don't talk about a patient with communication problems in her presence—it is demeaning and isolating.

Communication problems

A stroke can cause difficulties with communication and language (see p. 34). The patient may no longer understand the spoken and written word (receptive dysphasia) or be unable to express herself through speech or writing (motor dysphasia); on rare occasions, she may have problems with both understanding and expression. Some patients are unable to speak because the muscles used in speech are weak or paralyzed (dysarthria).

A speech therapist will assess the patient's needs while she is still in hospital and establish a treatment plan. Unfortunately, in some places, there are too few speech therapists to give the intensive, ongoing treatment some patients need. This makes it vital for carers and friends to help as much as possible. Ask the speech therapist exactly what the problem is and what you can do to help recovery.

Helping with receptive dysphasia

◆ Speak clearly and simply in short sentences and allow time for the patient to understand what you have said.

◆ Repeat yourself if she hasn't understood.

◆ Use everyday phrases, such as "would you like a cup of tea?", and gesture or mime at the same time.

◆ If reading is affected, find picture books, magazines or comics with simple captions. Avoid children's publications if possible, although these may be all that are available.

◆ Encourage attempts at reading the headlines in the newspaper or a favourite magazine.

Helping with motor dysphasia

◆ Always talk naturally and normally, because the patient can understand as much as she did before the stroke.

◆ Encourage her to name everyday household objects.

LINES OF COMMUNICATION

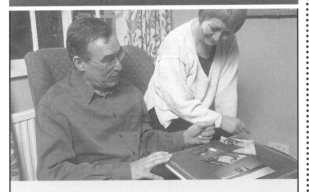

Looking at pictures and photographs of familiar objects and places and encouraging the patient to name them can help to overcome motor dysphasia.

3

YOU REALLY NEED TO KNOW

◆ Being unable to communicate is frustrating and isolating, and trying to make yourself understood can be exhausting and enraging. Encourage the patient to practise a little at a time and to try to stay calm.

◆ Do not shout, talk down or use childish language when communicating with a stroke patient.

◆ Read with the patient as well as encouraging her to read on her own.

◆ Listen carefully to what the patient says then tell her what you think she meant, to demonstrate success.

◆ Suggest she makes gestures or draws simple pictures to help her communicate.

◆ Encourage her to practise simple handwriting.

◆ Have pen and paper close at hand as many patients are able to write down what they mean before they regain the ability to express ideas in speech.

Helping with dysarthria

◆ Treatment focuses on regaining the ability to use the muscles that control speech. The carer and patient should practise the exercises set by the speech therapist together every day.

Possible problems

Ten percent of stroke patients suffer a second stroke within the first year. After a year the chances of a second stroke reduce further.

Sensible precautions

Even though most stroke patients do not have a second stroke, their risk of having one is higher than that of someone who has never had a stroke, and the likelihood of a second stroke increases if the patient does not take sensible precautions. These include changes to diet and lifestyle (see p. 50), sticking faithfully to any programme of medication and having regular check-ups. The physical and mental effects of a stroke may make it difficult for a patient to do all this without outside help, so the carer's role is vital.

Taking the medication

A variety of drugs are used to combat the root causes of strokes (see p. 28), and they are sometimes given in combinations. The confusion that is common in the first few days after a stroke can make it difficult for both patient and carer to grasp fully what has to be taken

KEEPING AN EYE ON PROGRESS

High blood pressure is usually symptomless and it also tends to rise with age. Both of these factors make it vital that a stroke patient's blood pressure is measured at regular intervals to monitor the effectiveness of the drug treatment and lifestyle changes. It is likely that once the patient has been prescribed medication to lower high blood pressure, she will have to take it for the rest of her life. Blood samples may be taken to check blood cholesterol—high levels of which contribute to atherosclerosis—and levels of anticoagulant drugs.

when, and why. The answer is to write out a list and organize a routine. This is important because some drugs, such as warfarin, must be taken at the same time each day. Ask the family doctor to check the list and routine, and take the opportunity to find out exactly what each drug does. Ask about possible side effects—not all drugs suit everybody, and if an individual patient does experience side effects it may be possible to take something different. Once you have settled into a routine, keep to it. Do not reduce dosages or leave out any drugs unless advised to do so by the doctor.

Routine check-ups

It is important for the family doctor to check the patient's condition on a regular basis. How often depends on the severity of the stroke and its effects. Contact your surgery if a series of appointments has not been set up for the patient. A check-up is also an opportunity for the doctor to monitor how rehabilitation is progressing and to discuss any side effects of medication.

Warning signs

There are very few warning signs that another stroke may be imminent, as high blood pressure does not usually cause any symptoms. However, a TIA (see p. 14) is a good indicator that another stroke may be about to occur. Symptoms of an attack can vary in severity and may last anything from a minute or two to 24 hours. The symptoms include any type of temporary weakness, lack of feeling, clumsiness or incapacity in any part of the body, as well as in speech and vision. If you have reason to suspect the patient has had a TIA, call the doctor without delay.

**YOU REALLY
NEED TO KNOW**

◆ Various different combinations of drugs may be prescribed, and some of them may have to be taken at the same time each day. Establish a routine and stick to it.

◆ Call the doctor immediately if you have reason to suspect that a stroke patient has had a TIA.

Possible problems

Chapter

4

DAY TO DAY
CARING

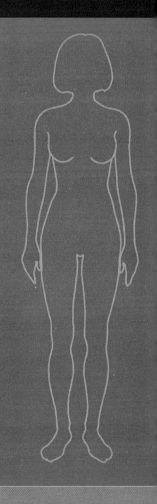

Being a carer

SELF-HELP

Get advice about the practicalities of being a carer and the possibilities for help from the Carers National Association, which has local branches throughout the country.

Life as a carer is far from easy. Once you have got over the inevitable shock you feel when a loved one suffers a stroke, worries about the future start to surface. For example, what are the prospects of recovery? Do I have the physical and mental strength to cope with long-term care? What sort of financial position will we be in? What support can I expect to get from other people? The first answers will come during the initial stay in hospital.

Problems to expect

The first few days after a stroke are a time of turmoil and distress and it can be difficult to take in and remember information. The following suggestions may help:

◆ Make lists of the questions you want to ask and write down the answers in some detail. Make sure you keep any leaflets you are given.

QUESTIONS TO ASK YOURSELF

◆ What are the financial implications if neither you nor the patient works and what benefits are available? (see p. 66)

◆ What support can you expect in the home? (see p. 68)

◆ Can you cope with any change of roles within the family? For example, can you take over what were the patient's chores or tasks?

◆ Can you cope with the demands of a strict routine, yet be flexible enough to change it as the patient regains his abilities?

◆ Do you have the physical strength and stamina to help the patient with everyday tasks and to help him regain his mobility? (see p. 42)

◆ Do you have the psychological strength to cope with the feelings of frustration, anger and guilt (see p. 56)—yours as well as those of the patient?

◆ Can you stay calm and be firm, patient, encouraging and positive?

◆ Learn as much as you can about the causes and effects of strokes, what has happened in the patient's particular case, and what the implications are. Above all, what is the outlook for the patient's recovery? (Bear in mind that it is hard for medical staff to make an exact prediction about this.)

◆ Ask the medical team for details of the drug regime and any dietary changes required.

◆ Ask about rehabilitation therapy and how you can help with this (see p. 32).

◆ Meet the occupational therapist and social worker (see p. 40) to organize any changes to the home and work out a care plan.

◆ Check the arrangements for discharge from hospital and for outpatient or home treatments.

The demands on you

The amount of care the patient will need depends on the severity of his stroke. Some patients need full-time care for several months or longer. When considering how you will cope, there are some important questions you should ask yourself (see chart).

Making a decision

Asking yourself difficult questions such as these is not being negative, but realistic. While caring can be very rewarding, it is also extremely demanding. Not everyone has the capability to be a full-time carer, and the most important thing is that the patient recovers as quickly as possible. Part-time caring, with support from others, may be the solution. Talk things through with the patient (if he is well enough), the family doctor, social worker and outside agencies (see p. 68) before deciding what to do.

YOU REALLY NEED TO KNOW

◆ After a stroke, people need different levels and duration of care, and being a carer can be very demanding.

◆ Establish what problems you are likely to face and how much help you are likely to receive.

◆ Talk things through with the support services before you decide how much you can do.

Being a carer

Finances and benefits

All disabled people are entitled to an assessment by social services to determine what financial and practical support is needed.

Get in touch with social services straight away if the patient has not been assessed.

If you are responsible for a major part of caring you should ask for a carer's assessment.

Financial considerations often cause great anxiety for both the stroke patient and her carer. They also play an important part in the carer's decision about the level of care he can provide. The problem is made worse if the patient previously looked after the family's finances and can now no longer do so. If the patient was working before her stroke, you must face up to reality and ask yourself how long it will be before she can work again, or if work will ever be possible again. If you work, can you afford to give up your job completely or take a prolonged leave of absence?

Work out your financial position

The first thing to do is sit down and take stock of the financial situation—you will need this information when you discuss benefits and the practical support available with social services.

Many stroke patients and their carers are elderly and have a set income from a retirement pension. Unfortunately, having a disability costs money: heating bills are higher, and special aids, home adaptations and domestic help all come at a price. Depending on your circumstances, you may be eligible for a subsidy or you may not have to pay at all, and in most cases, extra benefits will be available.

The situation is different for carers who have a job. If you can, delay any decision to give up your job until you know how long your responsibilities as a carer will last. Ask for a leave of absence—unpaid if necessary—instead. Later on, you may be able to get a part-time job (see p. 68) if full-time work is not possible. A part-time job will not only help with the finances, it will also restore some of your independence and social contact.

Find out about benefits

Ask social services or the Benefits Agency to give you details about all the financial help that is available, both to the patient and to you as the carer. The level of some of the benefits listed in the chart below varies according to the assessment of your financial situation.

WHAT BENEFITS ARE AVAILABLE?

◆ Attendance Allowance and Continual Attendance Allowance—paid weekly by social services to the patient if she needs either full-time or part-time care. It is not means-tested.

◆ Disability Living Allowance—paid tax-free to a patient under the age of 65 who requires extra help with day-to-day care and/or transport.

◆ Incapacity Benefit—paid to people under 65 who cannot work because of disability or sickness. A medical certificate is required.

◆ Invalid Care Allowance—paid to the carer as a weekly benefit. This is means-tested and is not available to anyone who has even a small income (at the time of writing, only £50 per week after certain deductions).

◆ Home Responsibilities Protection—awarded to individuals below retirement age who do not work in order to be carers, to ensure that they receive their full State Retirement Pension in the future.

◆ Housing grants—to adapt the home to make it suitable for the disabled person.

◆ VAT exemptions—certain items for the disabled can be bought tax-free at "disabled living centres" (see p. 78).

(see p. 78)

YOU REALLY NEED TO KNOW

◆ A stroke plays havoc with the finances of both the patient and her carer, whether or not she was working before it happened.

◆ Make sure you know what your entitlements are and that you receive all the financial help available to reduce money worries and improve the quality of life for all concerned.

Finances and benefits

Support for carers

SELF-HELP

✓ Your local community health council (CHC) can provide information about all NHS health services, and is also the body to turn to if you have any complaints.

✓ Some people with communication problems find that a personal computer helps. Contact AbilityNet (formerly The Foundation for Communication for the Disabled, see p. 78) for more information.

In theory, there is a considerable amount of support available to carers, but in practice, what can actually be obtained varies from one part of the country to another. Social services co-ordinate provision of basic support, but there are a number of voluntary organizations that also have much to offer. Contact the Carers National Association and The Stroke Association for more details (see p. 78). Depending on individual circumstances, a charge—or a contribution to the costs—may be made for some support services.

Support in the home

There are two types of home support available for carers. The first is concerned with teaching the carer how to deal with the practicalities of caring for someone: moving the patient, washing him, helping him with the toilet and bathing, practising rehabilitation exercises and

A CARER'S ASSESSMENT

◆ If you provide a major part of a stroke patient's care, you are entitled to ask social services to take your views into account when they are deciding what support will be provided to the patient—this procedure is called a Carer's Assessment. In some areas, support is also provided specifically for the carer.

◆ If your circumstances or those of the patient change, ask social services to carry out a review of the situation— a review should in any case be carried out every so often as a matter of routine.

so on. This is normally the district nurse's responsibility, although in some areas a hospital-based liaison nurse may also play a part.

The second type of support is aimed at helping the carer more directly. In "respite care", a trained carer or volunteer takes over from the primary carer for a few hours or longer to give her a break. Again, what is available varies from area to area, but ask social services, the Carers National Association and The Stroke Association about the following services and voluntary organizations:

◆ home care and home help (social services)

◆ meals on wheels (social services)

◆ respite care in the home (Crossroads, through Carers National Association)

◆ help with the various different communication problems (see p. 58—Dysphasia Support, through The Stroke Association)

◆ longer-term respite care (see p. 74).

Support outside the home

Support given outside the home has two purposes: first, to give the carer a break from full-time caring and allow her to get on with everyday activities and, sometimes, to work part time; and second, to encourage the stroke patient to socialize and start to lead an active, more independent life once more. There is a range of options available, and you may want to investigate whether some or all of the following are available locally:

◆ day care centres (social services)

◆ carers' centres and lunch clubs (Carers National Association)

◆ stroke clubs (The Stroke Association).

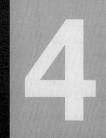

Support for carers

Family and friends

DO's AND DONT's

✓ Do keep family and friends informed about the patient's problems and any progress being made.

✗ Don't exclude the grandchildren. Children are often more adaptable than adults and are usually willing to spend plenty of time with their grandparents, perhaps playing cards or doing a jigsaw.

While expert help and advice can go a long way toward reducing the demands that are inevitably placed on a carer, you should never underestimate the warmth, reassurance, support and practical help that family and friends can also offer.

It is easy for the main carer to fall into the trap of being so keen to cope single-handedly that other people—especially family and friends—feel unwanted and excluded and, in the belief that all is well, soon stop offering to help. Ultimately, though, this attitude helps neither the carer nor the patient: the carer becomes increasingly tired, both physically and mentally, while the patient suffers from a lack of mental stimulation and her rehabilitation starts to suffer.

It is easier, too, for all concerned, if family members and friends understand the problems a stroke patient is experiencing, come to terms with the inevitable changes

KEEPING IN TOUCH

Caring for a stroke patient can take up a considerable amount of time and it is easy to let relationships with family and friends slide. But it is important to both carer and patient to make time to keep up these relationships. And amidst all the upheaval that inevitably follows a stroke, friends and family members—especially children and grandchildren—often need to know that they are still loved by both of you.

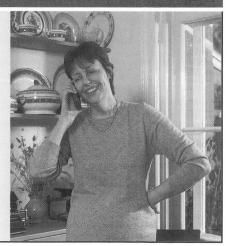

and together go through what can be almost a grieving process that may involve resentment, anger and guilt.

Accepting help

At first, you may feel that you can cope on your own. But as the cumulative effect of single-handed caring takes its toll, and depending on the severity of the stroke, you may find yourself unable to continue. Unfortunately, it often happens that if you refuse help in the early days it is not offered again, because people assume that you are coping. Rising to the challenge can be satisfying at first, but as time goes by you may feel resentment that people around you do not notice your exhaustion and need for a break. Instead they carry on with their own lives, reassured that you seem to be managing perfectly well on your own.

Practical help can take many forms, whether with day-to-day care, rehabilitation, household chores, shopping, cooking meals, gardening or going on outings. From the carer's point of view, the important thing is to take advantage of offers of help and use the free time to do what you want—above all don't hover nearby to check that your helpers can cope.

Help with speech therapy

A circle of willing friends and relatives is particularly important when a stroke patient has any form of communication problem (see p. 58). It is almost impossible for a carer to provide enough opportunities to practise skills in a social context single-handedly. But, with the guidance of a speech therapist or a dysphasic support group (see p. 78), family and friends can play a major role in rehabilitation.

(see p. 58) ... (see p. 78)

YOU REALLY NEED TO KNOW

◆ Caring for a stroke victim can be both physically and mentally exhausting. Do not be a martyr—accept all the help that is offered and if it is not forthcoming, ask for it.

◆ Family and friends can be particularly helpful when a stroke victim suffers from communication problems.

Family and friends

Looking after yourself

Physical and mental exhaustion affect everyone's health, no matter how strong their constitution. It is vital that carers look after themselves, not only for their own sake, but for that of the patient too.

The physical and emotional demands of caring for a stroke patient make it all too easy for the carer to forget to look after herself. But if you fall ill, the patient will suffer too, because he might have to go back into hospital or move into a nursing home if no other full-time carer is available. Some patients can be very demanding, and expect their requests to be satisfied immediately, expressing frustration and anger when this doesn't happen. In such cases it may be necessary for you—or the family doctor or district nurse—to point out the possible consequences if your own health suffers.

A healthy body...

Pay attention to the following to keep you in good physical condition:

◆ Plenty of sleep—you will probably need more sleep than you did before because of the physical demands

LOOK OUT FOR THE DANGER SIGNS

Talk things over with your doctor if you notice any of the following signs that things are getting too much for you:

◆ unusual or frequent muscular aches and pains

◆ tiredness and insomnia

◆ increased irritability and a short temper

◆ loss of appetite

◆ a tendency to ignore the patient or treat him like a child or a nuisance

◆ failure to tackle everyday chores that you took in your stride previously

◆ anxiety

◆ reclusiveness and a lack of desire to go out and see other people

being made on you. If you can't spend longer in bed, set time aside for a nap during the day.

◆ A good diet—including five helpings of fresh fruit and vegetables a day as well as protein, fibre and carbohydrate.

◆ Fresh air and exercise—try for three half-hour sessions of exercise, such as walking or swimming, a week.

...and a healthy mind

Psychological and emotional well-being are important for physical and mental health, so follow these simple rules.

◆ Make time for yourself—organize each day so that there are periods in which you can be alone, even if it is only two half-hour spells a day. Don't use this time for chores—take a relaxing bath, read or sit in the garden. Only break this routine in an emergency.

◆ Communicate—make sure you have someone to talk things through with and discuss any problems and concerns. Make sure you don't become isolated—keep up links with family and friends on a daily basis. Use a break to chat with a friend on the telephone, and ask people round to see you—perhaps when the patient also has a visitor. Ask your family round for a meal—you could even ask them to bring it with them! Write letters or notes to people—receiving letters and cards back is a great boost to morale.

◆ Learn to relax—this plays an important part in reducing stress and increasing mental fitness. Read one of the many books on relaxation techniques or attend a course. There are some courses that are run specially for carers—contact the Carers National Association to see if there is one in your area.

◆ Socialize—make sure you keep up your social life outside the home (see p. 74).

YOU REALLY NEED TO KNOW

◆ It is essential that you take positive steps to safeguard your health when caring for a stroke patient. Consult your doctor straightaway if you think things are getting too much for you, either physically or emotionally.

◆ Smoking and drinking alcohol may reduce stress in the short term, but they can actually make the problem worse. Give up smoking and keep alcohol consumption to moderate levels.

Looking after yourself

Looking after yourself

It is a mistake to fall into the trap of thinking that you have to give up everything to care for a stroke patient. Doing so helps neither you nor the patient.

Taking time for yourself

No one can care for a severely disabled patient 24 hours a day, 365 days a year. Any attempt to do so will take a heavy toll on the carer's physical and mental well-being, which in turn will reduce the patient's chances of successful rehabilitation. The general rule is that a carer should have one day, or two half-days, off each week and take at least two weeks' holiday a year. Respite care (see p. 69) is available to help you do this.

Even those caring for stroke patients with less severe disabilities need time to themselves, so that they can feel they are continuing to live their own lives. But one of the problems of being a carer is that taking a

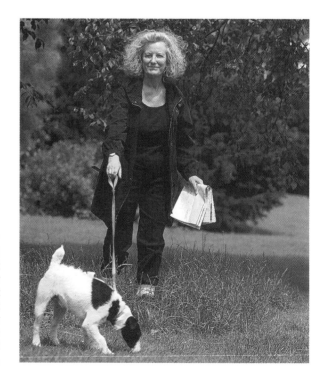

When you feel physically exhausted, it is tempting to use your leisure time to rest, but making the effort to get out into the fresh air may leave you no more physically tired, but mentally invigorated.

break, no matter how short, usually needs to be planned in advance. This is where social services and voluntary organizations (see p. 69) come in, along with your network of family and friends (see p. 70).

It is important that carers keep up their activities, interests and friendships, not only because it can be hard to pick up the threads once the patient has been rehabilitated, but also because meeting other people and concentrating on other activities can be a welcome distraction from the situation at home.

Try to establish a weekly routine with one day or, better, two half-days, free. Whether the patient visits a day-care centre, or an alternative carer comes to the home, it is important that you make the most of your opportunities.

Longer-term breaks

Being a carer is like having a full-time, demanding job—and one that continues at weekends. But, as with any job, it is important to have periods away so you can start again refreshed and with a renewed commitment.

For a weekend break, you may be able to arrange for a carer from a voluntary organization, such as Crossroads, to come and stay in the patient's home. For a longer holiday, however, the only solution may be a residential or nursing home. Depending on where you live, and your financial situation, you may be able to arrange this through social services. Voluntary organizations may also be able to help (see p. 78).

It can be difficult for a stroke patient to come to terms with having to go into a nursing home, as there is often an understandable fear of abandonment and reluctance to meet new people. Explain why you need a break and reassure him that this is a short-term measure.

Looking after yourself

Understanding the jargon

Many of the terms you will meet when finding out more about the causes and effects of a stroke may be unfamiliar to you. This page gives some definitions,and on page 78 you will find addresses of useful contact groups.

ANEURYSM—a localized swelling of the inner wall of an artery that has been weakened by atherosclerosis (see below). It may rupture through the outer wall of the artery, causing a haemorrhage

ARTERIOSCLEROSIS—a progressive thickening, hardening and so narrowing of the arteries—blood pressure must increase to force blood through them

ATHEROSCLEROSIS—narrowing of arteries caused by deposits of cholesterol (a fatty substance) in their walls. It is the commonest form of arteriosclerosis

CEREBELLUM—the area of the brain that controls co-ordination, balance and posture

CEREBRAL ARTERIES—the four main arteries that supply the brain with oxygenated blood. Two travel up the back of the neck and two up the front, joining at the base of the brain in a circle

CEREBRAL HEMISPHERES—the largest part of the brain, the two cerebral hemispheres receive sensory information from the rest of the body in specific control centres and initiate action

CEREBRAL OEDEMA—swelling of the brain tissues as a result of bleeding, trauma or the death of brain cells. It increases pressure within the skull

CEREBROVASCULAR ACCIDENT (CVA)—the blockage of or disruption to the blood supply to the brain (ie, a stroke)

DYSARTHRIA—difficulty with speech when a stroke has damaged the brain's control centre for the throat and mouth muscles

DYSPHASIA—difficulty in understanding speech and writing (sensory dysphasia) or in communicating through speech and writing (motor dysphasia) as a result of damage to brain control centres

EMBOLUS—foreign matter in the blood that may become lodged in a blood vessel and cause a stroke

HEMIPLEGIA—paralysis of one side of the body

HYPERTONIC—overcontracted or spastic (of muscle)

HYPOTONIC—lacking tone (of muscle)

ISCHAEMIA—an area of the body that has no blood supply due to some blockage of the circulation

MULTIPLE INFARCTS—repeated very small strokes whose effects are similar to Alzheimer's disease

SUBARACHNOID HAEMORRHAGE—bleeding into the space between the membranes lining the brain

THROMBUS—a clot of blood in an artery that has been narrowed and may break away to form an embolus (see above)

TRANSIENT ISCHAEMIC ATTACK (TIA)—a stroke whose symptoms clear completely within 24 hours

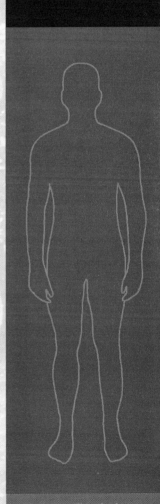

Understanding the jargon

Useful addresses

THE STROKE ASSOCIATION
Stroke House
Whitecross Street
London EC1Y 8JJ
Advisory Line: 020 7566 0330
Publish a wide range of leaflets.
Contact them for details of local
clubs throughout the UK

DIFFERENT STROKES
Sir Walter Scott House
PO Box 5082
Milton Keynes MK5 7ZH
Tel: 01908 236033
For people under 60 who have
suffered a stroke and their carers

DISABLED LIVING FOUNDATION
380-384 Harrow Road
London W9 2HU
Tel: 020 7289 6111
Helpline: 0870 603 9177
Contact them for advice on specialist
aids and adaptations to make
everyday tasks easier

CARERS NATIONAL ASSOCIATION
20-25 Glasshouse Yard
London EC1A 4JT
Tel: 020 7490 8818
Carers Line: 0808 808 7777

ASSOCIATION OF CROSSROADS CARE
10 Regent Place
Rugby CV21 2PN
Tel: 01788 573653
Provides respite care in the home

ACTION FOR DYSPHASIC ADULTS
1 Royal Street
London SE1 7LL
Tel: 020 7261 9572

AGE CONCERN ENGLAND
1268 London Road
London SW16 4ER
Tel: 0800 7314931
Gives general advice on caring
for an older person

ABILITYNET
Helpline: 0800 269545
www.abilitynet.co.uk

Index

Index

Acknowledgements
Photographs: Corbis 28; Sally & Richard Greenhill 27, 62-3; Science Photo Library 60; (A B Dowsett) 16-17, 24-5, 64, 72; (Simon Fraser/Brampton Day Hospital, Cumbria) 32; (Hexham General) 56; (John Greim) 22-3; (Will & Deni McIntyre) 31; (Prof. P Motta) 7, 41, 76-7; (Larry Mulvehill) 21; (Sheila Terry) 51; (Ed Young) 35; Sidhilcare 46.
All other photographs by Guglielmo Galvin.

Edited and designed by Phoebus Editions, 72-80 Leather Lane, London EC1N 7TR

Special thanks to Mike Newby and Vickie Walters for for agreeing to model for the photographs. Thanks also to the Disabled Living Foundation for the loan of aids for photography. Tel. 020 7289 6111 for more information on products.